# *AN INSIDE JOB* Companion

# Making Healing Personal

SUSAN BARBARA APOLLON

*An Inside Job Companion: Making Healing Personal*
is a workbook that accompanies
*An Inside Job: A Psychologist Shares Healing Wisdom
for Your Cancer Journey,*
by Susan Apollon

**To order copies of *An Inside Job* or
*An Inside Job Companion*,
please visit www.aninsidejobforhealingcancer.com**

Copyright © 2017 Susan Barbara Apollon

All rights reserved.

Published by:
Matters of the Soul, LLC
Box 403
Yardley, PA 19067

ISBN: 978-0-9754036-1-7

Library of Congress Control Number: 2017901930

The stories referred to in this book are true. However, names and identifying details have been changed to protect the privacy of all concerned (except for a few who have given permission to use their names).

All rights reserved. No part of this book may be used or reproduced in any form or by any means, or stored in a database or retrieval system without the prior written permission of the publisher, except in the case of brief quotations embodied in critical articles or reviews. Making copies of any part of this book for any purpose other than your own personal use is a violation of United States copyright laws.

Printed in the United States of America

I dedicate *An Inside Job Companion: Making Healing Personal* to each of you who have read *An Inside Job* in your quest for healing wisdom. It is my wish that the following exercises help you gain a richer understanding of the energetic dynamics available to you for harnessing a healthy immune system, as well as a deeper understanding of the nature of healing. You have my loving support on this challenging journey.

# Acknowledgments

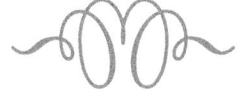

Thank you to each of you who have taken your precious time and energy to read *An Inside Job*, and who wish to internalize and apply these guiding principles to assist the healing capacity of your body. This book is written for you, with the hope that it will further empower, inform, educate, and inspire you on your unique healing journey.

The very existence of this workbook and the book that birthed it rests with the crew at DeHart and Company—including Dottie DeHart, Eve Campbell, Anna Campbell, Meghan Waters, Ashley Lamb, Paige Hendren, Megan Brendle, Brad Metzgar, and Kory Bailey. I will always be grateful for your loving dedication to this project, for your inspiration, perseverance, and your vision of the impact this pair of books will have on those who incorporate the material into their lives. Each of you holds a special place in my heart. Thank you again and again for all you are and all you do for me and for those in need of this material. I can't thank you enough for always being there for me, for everything!

Thank you, Warren, for having been so lovingly patient with me on this journey of creating both the book, *An Inside Job*, and *An Inside Job Companion*. None of this would have been possible without your loving support and all you do to enrich my life. My heart always overflows with love for you.

# Introduction

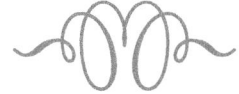

I am honored that you have chosen *An Inside Job* as worthy of your precious time and energy along your healing journey. In writing this book, I wanted to give you the best of what I have learned in working with those challenged by an illness—including cancer—to help you cope with this overwhelming experience, and help you navigate the major decisions you must make.

After finishing the manuscript for *An Inside Job*, I suddenly realized that in order to truly assist and guide you, there was one more element I could offer you. I wanted to help you focus in on those significant points that need to be integrated into your life and perspective, and to help you become aware of how your world view shapes and impacts your wellness. Finally, I want you to recognize that the lessons in this workbook apply to anyone seeking guidance on how to stay whole, balanced, and well—no matter what trials you are facing.

You may be wondering how to get the most out of *An Inside Job Companion: Making Healing Personal.* I believe in practicing KIS (keeping it simple), and I hope you will follow suit as you approach each upcoming exercise. I chose to go back through *An Inside Job* chapter by chapter and determine which tools and points I felt warranted your additional reflection and attention. Always know, there are no right or wrong answers—only how you feel about and view your challenge.

I also encourage you to reflect on these exercises and journal on your own, but, additionally, do consider asking a few friends or those dealing with similar circumstances to join you in discussing your perspective, thoughts, and what you, personally, are learning from your journey. I promise you that whether you complete these exercises solo or as an integral part of a community or group, you will find yourself feeling better, more empowered, more confident, and—believe it or not—even more at peace with your situation. The goal: healing in the form of peace and an increased sense of balance and wholeness. Enjoy!

# Working with Energy and Vibrations

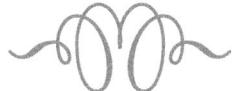

Energy is everything. You, as well as everything you see, touch, and feel, are made of energy. Further, the quality of your vibrations determines how good or bad you feel. With this understanding in mind, describe times in your life when you were energetically and vibrationally very "low"—almost unable to function normally—and when you were truly happy and at peace, thus vibrating at a "high" level.

Can you recall some of your thoughts during each of these times? For example, when your vibrations were very low, you may have thought something like, *I do not feel like doing anything. I can't do much. My heart feels broken. I wish things were better at home/in my marriage/at work.* When feeling joyful and vibrating at a higher level, thoughts may include: *At this moment I feel wonderful, happy, motivated, empowered, and like I can do anything! Everything is going well with the kids/at work/at school/at home.*

# Staying Stressed and Sick

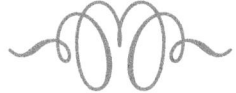

Stress and illness often go hand in hand. (Usually, one follows the other!) Give examples that validate the relationship between stress and illness in your life.

# Understanding the Factors that Influence Your Energy

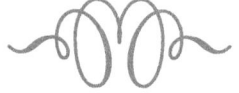

What factors and aspects of your life (such as personal, professional, spiritual, financial, and lifestyle-related) contribute to your feeling energetically alive, content, and connected to your essence and to others?

# What Is Causing Your Disconnection?

What factors contribute to your energetically experiencing a sense of disconnection from who you are and from life itself (including anything or anyone you currently grieve, miss, or have lost in any aspect of your life)?

# Discovering and Choosing Self-Love

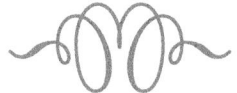

What does self-love mean to you? How can your immune system's 60 trillion cells experience self-love? What makes them know and feel they are loved? List several ways you can practice self-love today. Keep in mind that many methods are free and easy, such as taking a bubble bath, a quiet stroll in a park, or enjoying some relaxing music.

# Find Personalized Methods to Release Pain

What do you feel you need to do to release and let go of the regrets, anger, and negative thoughts to which you are attached and which have been keeping you from moving on with your life? (Some methods may include journaling, affirmations, visualizations, a new choice, intentions, seeking clarity, surrendering, adopting a "just do it" attitude, etc.)

# Learning to Restore Balance and Peace

Think of times when you experienced healing (the restoration of balance and peace) in the past. Consider the choices you made to achieve this (your thoughts, activities, intentions, etc.) and write about how you can use these same methods to initiate healing today.

# Understanding the Bliss-Healing Connection

What does following your passion have to do with healing (in terms of your understanding of energy)? Do you notice a difference in your energy levels when you have spent time doing something you love, like dancing, drawing, or singing?

# Finding Compassion and Love for the Difficult People in Your Life

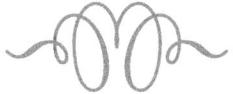

Think of someone in your life who has been challenging—if not purely difficult—and represents resistance for you. Then, imagine that person not being in your life. Allow yourself to fill with compassion and love for them. Consider who you would be had you not had this person as part of your journey. Be conscious of your feelings and your thoughts. What *gifts* have they given you that have enabled you to become who you are today? (These may include resiliency, strength, self-knowledge, empowerment, curiosity, wisdom, knowing right from wrong, self-confidence, etc.) Imagine yourself expressing gratitude and appreciation to this individual for being in your life and enabling you to evolve as you have.

# Like Energy Attracts Like Energy

To better understand and experience the concept *like energy attracts like energy*, place your dominant hand on your heart and then, with eyes closed, bring to mind someone or something for whom or what you feel great love. Notice how you are feeling—and vibrating energetically. If *this* is your dominant vibration, you attract equally wonderful vibrations into your life. Now place your dominant hand on your heart, and, with eyes closed, bring to mind someone or something for whom you feel great negativity, pain, and/or suffering. If *this* is your dominant vibration, such a low vibratory experience attracts to you equivalently low vibratory experiences. Record your reflections in the space below.

# Stress Begets More Stress

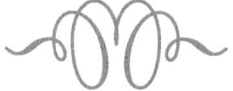

Can you think of a time or times in your life when you experienced continued stress and stress-related thoughts that were followed by a series of negative experiences? This phenomenon is indicative of the relationship between like-energy thoughts attracting like-energy experiences. It is how the universe works! Write about a time in your life in which your low vibrations and stress helped manifest ongoing negative situations. What can you learn from those experiences?

# Are You Living in Alignment with Your Core Values?

Think about your core values (regarding love, honesty, integrity, presence, kindness, loyalty, etc.) and then consider whether you are truly living in alignment with those values. Give a percentage to your current sense of alignment. This percentage is an indication of where you are energetically and vibrationally. The higher your energy and vibrations, the more at peace and less resistant you become. Peace is achieved when we choose to remove all resistance. (In this sense, "resistance" means pushing for or against something and trying to be in control.) How is your core value alignment, and what can you do to adjust it?

# Coping with Loss (and What You Can Learn from It)

Recall times of great loss in your life. What choices did you make that enabled you to energetically heal and feel lighter and better following a loss? What did you focus your energy on? How can your choices continue to foster healing as you face new challenges?

# Harnessing the Will to Live

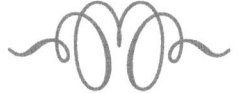

Humans possess a powerful force—the will to live—that drives them to survive traumas, strife, and adversity. When has your will to live seen you through difficult and challenging times? (You can include the present.) Can you think of someone whose will to live enabled them to live, and even thrive, despite their challenging illness?

# Identifying and Using the Guiding Principles for Healing

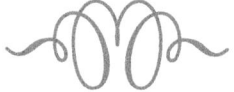

"Guiding Principles" refer to the beliefs we hold about our inherent ability to heal and thrive in the face of an illness. For example, understanding that *like energy attracts like energy* can guide your choices and your mindset during your cancer journey. What major guiding principles will you use to manage your life and your challenge with cancer or any life-threatening illness? Have these principles shifted since your diagnosis? If so, please explain further.

# Choosing an Uplifting Perspective

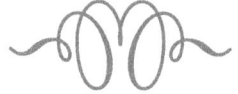

It is important to adopt the uplifting perspective that everything in life, including an illness such as cancer, is actually a teacher. Given this view, how has your perspective changed, if at all, since your diagnosis? Have you noticed that by choosing the gift of a positive perspective (for example, believing *life is a teacher* or *cancer is a gift*), or by surrendering your concerns to your Higher Power, you find yourself less angry, more in alignment with your values, and happier overall? Have you observed the opposite occurring when you hold onto negative viewpoints about life, people, and situations—and that these lead to a lack of well-being? Such is the power of shifting your thoughts. Likewise, focusing on something that feels good or not good influences the ability of your immune system to care for you.

# Could Cancer Be a Gift?

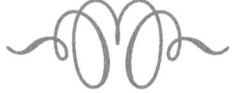

Remember that you have a choice in how you view your cancer diagnosis. What if you chose to view cancer as a gift instead of a horrible fate? What gifts or lessons has cancer taught you? Have you learned to let go, to forgive, to love yourself more fully? Have you learned what truly matters in life, as well as what doesn't matter? Record the gifts cancer has given you below and continue adding to this list as you recognize new blessings on your journey.

# Exploring Your Vital Role in Disappointing Situations

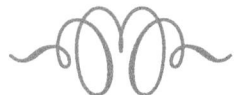

At times, we may lose sight of our power to create the lives we want for ourselves. It is important to remember that we continually help manifest our reality. Think of past situations you've hoped for that never manifested. In the space below, note what you were doing (or thinking) energetically at the time that may have contributed to the unwanted outcome you received.

# The Path to Healing (Many Aspects of Healing Are Under Your Control)

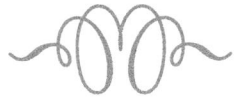

When have you experienced healing in your life? (Remember that healing can take many forms: physical, emotional, mental, or spiritual.) What factors contributed to your healing? How can you apply those factors to your current state of wellness?

# Can Spiritual Healing Occur Even When You Don't Heal Physically?

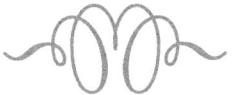

Consider the tremendous power of spiritual healing when one is physically ill. Think of those you know who did not heal physically from an illness, but nonetheless experienced a spiritual healing. What factors do you feel contributed to this transformation? How does a sense of peace and wellness (versus fear and turmoil) contribute to spiritual healing?

# How to Make Peace with Your Diagnosis

If you have cancer or a life-threatening illness, what do you see yourself doing to make peace (in other words, to *be* at peace) with your challenge? What emotions and needs should you release to find this sense of ease? (For example, you might release anger, resentment, the need to be in control, etc.) What actions might you experience and practice in order to have a peaceful quality of life? (Some examples might be unconditional love, patience, compassion, forgiveness, self-love, understanding, etc.)

# The Importance of Allowing Yourself to Grieve

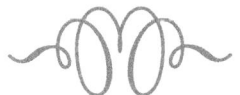

When you receive a diagnosis of cancer, what does it mean to you to allow yourself to grieve? Consider the factors that you may mourn the loss of: your previous state of health, your life roles and view of yourself, your identity, and your life as you knew it. Why does cancer represent a significant loss to you? Specifically, *what* do you grieve? How is your identity connected to your loss?

# Losses Bring Up Memories of Older Pain

Think of a recent or present loss you have experienced or currently face. Recall the feelings that arose when this loss occurred. What did the vibration of this loss remind you of and bring to the surface regarding past losses? Ask yourself, *What does this feeling I have now remind me of in relation to my past experiences with loss? How similar are the vibrations of both the past and the present? What do these similarities reveal?*

# Learning to Balance Your Grief

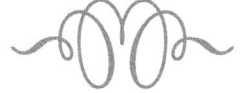

What do you do to balance your grief? What methods, tools, and activities do you engage in to balance your sadness, soothe your broken heart, and enable you to feel better? How can these tools be applied to grief surrounding your cancer diagnosis?

# Healing Exercise for Connecting to a Deceased Loved One or with Spirit

The following is an exercise to connect with a deceased loved one, Teacher, Guide, Angel, or your Source. The purpose of the exercise is to enable you to receive comfort, support, wisdom, and guidance—emotions and needs often experienced when we grieve someone or something we dearly miss and love.

Sit and allow yourself to focus on your breath inhalation and exhalation for a few moments. Allow yourself to move into a state of genuine relaxation. As you continue to focus on your breathing and your awareness of becoming more relaxed, choose to focus on one with whom you would like to connect. Sitting with a notebook and pen, request that, if they desire, they use you as a conduit to convey their thoughts to you. With pen in your dominant hand, while still relaxed, begin to write whatever comes to you. Let there be a free, automatic flow of thoughts coming through you. You may initiate a dialogue, asking questions, pausing, and then writing what you intuitively receive. There is a feeling of great comfort as we recognize that in the midst of our grieving our loss, we are not alone, after all.

# Exploring Face/Embrace/(Breathe)/Replace

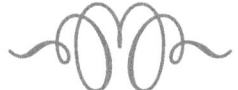

Face/Embrace/(Breathe)/Replace is an exercise that helps you intentionally identify and process your negative feelings rather than dwelling on them. Explain how Face/Embrace/(Breathe)/Replace may be considered a form of conscious grieving and how it can help you come to terms with illness. Notice that Breathe has been inserted here as a step to take following Embrace. The purpose is to consciously breathe in peace and consciously breathe out the thought that has caused you to feel your pain. Though it does not rhyme with Face, Embrace, Replace, it is a powerful step that enables you to release the thought that contributes to the blockage of your energetic healing. In the future, please think of this tool as Face/Embrace/(Breathe)/Replace.

*The following pages consist of a series of exercises, many of which are described in depth in An Inside Job. Play with the following crucial tools for healing whenever you can to align your spirit and process any unpleasant emotions you may be dealing with. The more often you try these exercises, the better adapted you become to taking control of your emotional and cognitive states—in other words, the better you feel! After experiencing each tool, take a moment or two to jot down your thoughts and observations.*

# Healing Tool #1: Use the SUDS Rating to Assess Your Emotion

Think of a situation or circumstance in which you feel anxious, fearful, and/or worried. Close your eyes, breathe deeply, scan your body, and rate the level of your emotion on a scale of 1-10 (with 10 being the highest). This is called a SUDS rating (Subjective Units of Distress Scale). It will help you assess the level of emotional distress (or lack thereof) you may be feeling and can become a catalyst for choosing a healthier alternative instead. Write your thoughts surrounding the emotions you encounter in the space below.

# Healing Tool #2: Face/Embrace/ (Breathe)/Replace

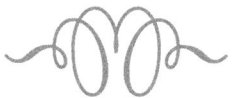

First, do a SUDS rating to assess your level of emotion. Practice the Face/Embrace/(Breathe)/Replace technique as described in *An Inside Job* for at least three to five minutes or more. When finished, close your eyes, breathe deeply again, and rate your level of emotion. Notice the power of the SUDS tool in helping you to decrease your emotional distress. Do this several more times until you have significantly reduced the level of your emotion.

# Healing Tool #3: The ABCs

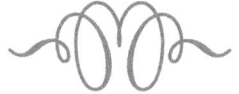

Do a SUDS rating to assess your level of emotion. Now, practice the ABCs tool as described in *An Inside Job*. Be sure to rate your emotion after practicing the ABCs tool. Determine how this practice feels for you. Notice whether the ABCs technique resonates less, more, or the same as the similar tool, Face/Embrace/(Breathe)/Replace. You may find that one technique feels more comfortable for you.

# Healing Tool #4: Mindfulness

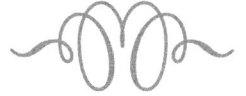

When you find yourself unable to stop focusing on a worry, fear, or concern, consider practicing the Mindfulness tool, as described in *An Inside Job*. It consists of the following steps: breathing in, observing and noticing, labeling (thought, feeling, sound, etc.), and finally detaching by breathing out. Any time you wish to release unpleasant emotions, repeat these steps for several minutes. Notice the increased sense of relaxation, peace, and well-being.

# Healing Tool #5: Tapping (The 10-10-90 Method)

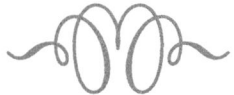

When you find yourself overwhelmed by troublesome thoughts and fears, close your eyes, scan your body, and rate your level of stress with a SUDS rating of 1-10 (with 10 being the highest). Then, start practicing the gamut tapping technique of 10-10-90. This is how you do it: Tap on the gamut of one hand while counting to 10. Stop tapping and count to 10. Now, resume tapping for about a minute and a half while breathing in and out. Then do the same on the other hand. This process equals one set. Do two more sets of the 10-10-90 (on each hand). A cycle equals three sets. After you have completed a cycle, do another SUDS rating. Do another cycle or two until your SUDS numbers are significantly decreased.

*The goal of each of these exercises is to enable you to recognize your own ability to take control of your personal power and feel more calmness, peace, and well-being. You can use any or all of these to empower yourself whenever needed. But remember, practice is essential.*

# Facing Your Fear of Death

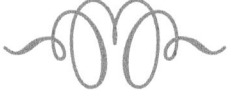

When facing an illness like cancer, you will likely experience frightening thoughts and anxieties centered around death. Given that we know energy does not die, but is transformed, how does this knowledge impact your thoughts and perspective about what happens when you die? Explore your thoughts in the space below.

# Exploring the Afterlife Through Stories and NDEs

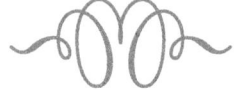

How have stories of life after life or near-death experiences influenced you and your perspective about life, death, and cancer? Do such stories enable you to think differently than you previously did? Do they inspire you and/or enable you to grow spiritually?

# Signs and Their Significance

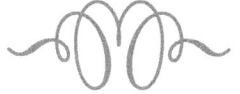

What do *signs* mean to you in relation to your experience with illness? Have you asked for—and received—any signs signaling you to feel peace and comfort? What meaning did you give these signs? How did they leave you feeling?

_____
_____
_____
_____
_____
_____
_____
_____
_____
_____
_____
_____
_____
_____
_____
_____

# Exploring Your Synchronicities

Share synchronicities from your own life that were too meaningful to simply be coincidences. Why were you so sure of their significance? How did or do these synchronicities help you to shift your belief system? Have any of your experiences significantly caused you to open your heart to the possibility of miracles?

_____

_____

_____

_____

_____

_____

_____

_____

_____

_____

_____

_____

_____

_____

# Receiving Otherworldly Comforts

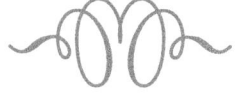

Describe an incident or incidents in your life (such as "Allie's Signs" or Linda's tale of angelic intervention as featured in *An Inside Job*) in which you personally experienced a sense of giving or receiving energy that was comforting and healing. What meaning can you take from these experiences?

# How Cancer Rearranges Your Priorities

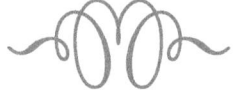

For many, cancer is a wakeup call that inspires swift change in people's lives. How has cancer shifted your priorities? Is there anything you will change about your life moving forward? In the space below, first list your priorities prior to your diagnosis. Then, write your new priority list. What are the biggest changes you notice?

# Seeking Sources of Peace Along Your Cancer Journey

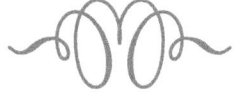

As you face a cancer diagnosis and undergo treatments, it is important to seek and maintain a sense of peace that will facilitate your wellness along the way. What specifically has helped you find peace on your health journey? Some examples might include inspiring messages, people, stories, books, and your beliefs.

# Understanding Your Higher Power

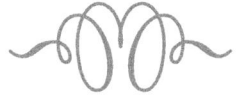

God, Source, Higher Power: Each of these expressions signifies the loving energy of the Universe. Please feel free to view the term "Higher Power" through your own belief system. What is *your* Higher Power? How can you connect to your Higher Power?

# Growing Your Spirit

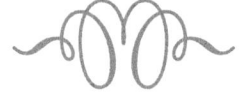

What does it mean to you to grow your spirit—and how does your Higher Power help in the growth of your spirit? How has the experience of cancer helped you grow your spirit? How has cancer helped connect you with your Higher Power?

# Your Personal Relationship with Spirituality

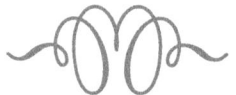

What does the term "spirituality" mean to you? What can you do to get more in touch with your spirituality?

# How Can You *Give* and *Be* Love?

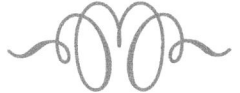

What do you believe it means to love unconditionally and to *be* love? How can you practice loving unconditionally (to yourself and others!)? In what ways can you *be* love? How does giving unconditional love and *being* love support your mind, body, and spirit as you face an illness?

# Enhancing the Power of Your Prayers

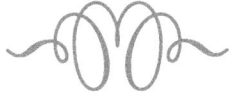

Prayer is a powerful way to nourish your spirit, and *An Inside Job* delves into ways to use prayer to connect to the divine and deepen your sense of peace. In the space provided, name three methods you have learned (and were not aware of) that enhance the power of your prayers. For example, the expectation *that your prayer has already been answered* allows you to dwell within a place of gratitude, which vibrationally raises your energy *as* you pray. If you have already put these suggestions into practice, please comment on your perspective regarding how this feels to you.

# The Body Temporarily Houses the Soul

In the space provided, explain what it means to be a soul in a physical body having a spiritual journey. How does this knowledge affect you vibrationally?

# Living by the Law of Attraction

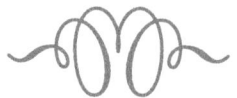

The Law of Attraction is the name given to the concept *like energy attracts like energy*. On the lines below, describe times in your life when the Law of Attraction contributed to creating your reality (for better or for worse).

# Realizing the Power of Your Words

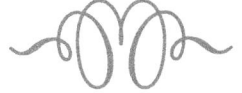

Regarding the Law of Attraction, discuss your perspective regarding the vibrational meaning of the words we choose to say to ourselves and others. How can your words affect your life?

# Shifting Your Thoughts to Facilitate Wellness

Provide examples of words (thoughts) you say to yourself that do not feel good. Describe and discuss how the unkind/unloving/unsupportive words you say to yourself affect you vibrationally. Realize that you must shift to feel better words, thoughts, and affirmations. Instead of negative thoughts and beliefs, what can you tell yourself that will empower you vibrationally?

_____

_____

_____

_____

_____

_____

_____

_____

_____

_____

# Harnessing the Power of Affirmations

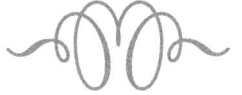

Affirmations are positive phrases you can use to influence how you feel about yourself and your circumstances. How can you use affirmations to empower yourself? How can they influence your healing journey? In the space below, list some affirmations you can use each day to stay in a place of peace, wellness, and gratitude.

# Exploring the Vital Connection Between Strength and Forgiveness

Consider Gandhi's quote, "The weak can never forgive. Forgiveness is the attribute of the strong." How do you currently see yourself regarding this quote? Are you able to forgive yourself and others or do you need to work on letting go of old grudges, losses, and letdowns? What would you have to change in order to forgive?

# Forgiveness Is an Act of Self-Love

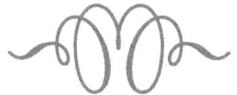

What does it mean to you to be both love (loving) and forgiving with yourself and with others? Describe how you feel—emotionally as well as physically—when you forgive yourself or someone else. How do you think forgiveness (and the resulting vibration of unconditional love) impacts your immune system?

# The Link Between Releasing the Past and Feeling Better

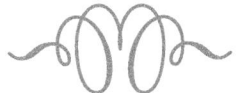

When you find yourself unable to let go of painful feelings or a painful event from the past, you deeply hinder your ability to heal. For your own peace of mind and healing, consider and write about any deeply upsetting situations and/or feelings that you have been unable to process, express, and release. While breathing in and out, imagine your release of each of these situations, along with their associated feelings and thoughts. Notice how you feel before and after doing this exercise. Be sure to follow this up with envisioning yourself filling up with love. Again, notice how you are now feeling.

# Learning the Power of "I Did My Best"

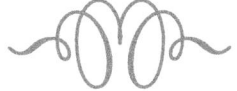

Practice integrating the words "I did my best" into your life every time you feel guilty, responsible, or in regard to situations when you could have done better. Describe specifically what you would like these words to help you heal.

# Create Your Forgiveness List

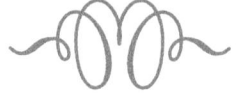

Remember that forgiving others benefits you as much as those you forgive; it is truly an expression of self-love. Besides yourself, who do you choose to forgive? In the space below, write a letter of forgiveness to one person you need to forgive. Affirm the written words of forgiveness in your soul.

# The Steep Price of Withholding Forgiveness

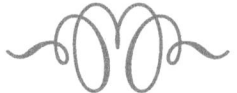

*An Inside Job* reveals the story of Sue Chance and features her book, *Stronger Than Death: When Suicide Touches Your Life.* Her son's suicide plunged Sue into an abyss of self-blame and despair. Only by finally forgiving herself as well as her son could Sue begin to find peace again. In the space below, answer the following question: How does NOT forgiving yourself and others hurt you?

# Work to Release Your Past

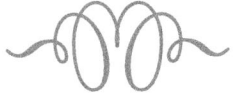

What do you need to forgive yourself for? Make a list in the space provided of everything you would like to release and forgive in your history. Then begin the work of releasing self-blame.

# Understanding the Harmony of Alignment

What does it mean to be in alignment with your heart or inner being?

# Assess Your Current Level of Alignment

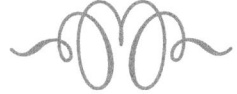

Do you feel out of alignment right now? What do you feel is contributing to your lack of alignment? What would you choose to release or change in order to create peace and alignment within you?

# Cancer's Role in Realigning Yourself

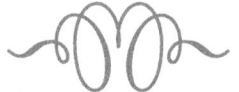

What has cancer taught you about your alignment? Has it clarified ways in which you might be living out of alignment? How has cancer expedited your healing journey?

# Exploring Tools for Alignment

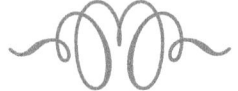

What tools can you choose to create alignment and peace within? Examples may include Donna Eden's Five Minute Energy Routine, focusing on the breath, saying "no" more often, practicing affirmations, etc. Choose exercises that resonate with you and bring you a sense of calm and connection to your spirit.

# Explore How the Breath Can Facilitate Healing

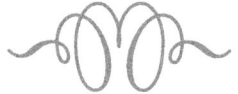

Mindful breathing exercises can help you find healing and balance along your journey. Take time to practice the "15-Minute Peace Plan" outlined in *An Inside Job* for several days (or up to a week). How does focused breathing and relaxation alter your levels of stress, pain, or unease? Jot down any changes you observe in your physiological, emotional, and mental responses as your stress diminishes. Note which changes made you feel more or less comfortable. For example, becoming very relaxed may be both peaceful and comfortable, as well as *uncomfortable* for those who are used to always doing and being active, rather than simply *being*.

# Acknowledge Miracles in Your Life

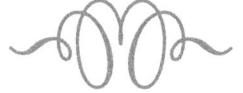

As you face illness and uncertainty, it is important to be open to the possibility of miracles and extraordinary experiences—and to ponder their significance. In the space provided, write about the times in your life in which you felt a miracle had occurred. Maybe a check arrived in the mail when you desperately needed extra money, or an opportunity appeared out of the blue that changed your life. (Remember also that synchronicities may be considered miracles.) How did you know you had experienced a miracle?

# Open Yourself to Miracles

How would modifying your perspective and your outlook on life help lead to miracles *in* your life? (Hint: It is all about vibration—*especially* the vibration of love.) In the space provided, list five ways you can shift your perspective, increase your vibrational energy, and welcome more miracles.

# Receive Guidance from Your Higher Power

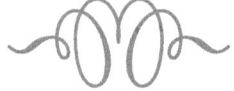

When blessed with the awareness that you have received guidance from your Higher Power, you can choose to either intuitively listen or not listen. But miracles and synchronicities happen when we choose to intuitively listen. For example, if you are going into surgery and are quietly talking to your deceased parents and then suddenly meet a nurse or doctor with your parent's name or see their name in print in front of you, you get to choose to either see this as a synchronicity and/ or a small miracle, or not. Describe those times when you sensed you had been comforted and/or guided by your Higher Power—perhaps your angels, God, or your Higher Self—which is connected to your Source.

# Understand the Importance of Family and Friends

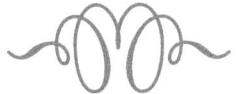

In the 1960s, it was discovered that the male residents of Roseto, PA, had significantly lower incidences of heart disease than the national average—even though they drank alcohol, smoked, and labored long days in the nearby quarries. Researchers soon concluded that the secret to the men's health was their sense of belonging within Roseto's tight-knit Italian-American community. In Roseto people felt cared for, family was emphasized, and relationships mattered. Sadly, over time, a shift in values sparked a decline in residents' health, and the incidence of heart disease eventually fell in line with the national average. Review the Roseto story as featured within *An Inside Job*. Consider how your lifestyle currently compares to that of the Roseto inhabitants—both before and after the studies occurred. Which lifestyle would you prefer? Can you see yourself incorporating the best of both worlds—or not?

# Identify Your Toxic Relationships

Do you have relationships that can be described as toxic? What do you feel makes them toxic? In the space provided, identify the relationships in your life that no longer "work." What can you do to improve these relationships? If you discover that—given your current circumstances—you can no longer participate in any of these relationships, what steps can you take to separate yourself and restore your sense of peace?

# What Is Holding You Back from Intimacy?

No matter your level of health, everyone needs intimacy—whether platonic or romantic. However, many people facing cancer have feelings of conflict surrounding the topic of intimacy. What fears do you have that get in the way of being more intimate with loved ones, family, and friends?

# Fostering the Healing Power of Intimacy

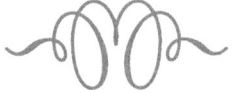

Engaging in frequent intimacy can be extremely healing. Make a point to bring more intimacy into every area of your life. What interventions can you see yourself engaging in to enable you to be more intimate? Some great examples are: cuddling with your pet, playing with your child/nephew/niece/grandchild, praying with your partner.

# Identifying Your Needs

Remember that your needs are important and that you have a right to communicate those needs to your friends and family. In the space below, list any needs that you wish to convey to your loved ones. Some examples might be: *I still need to feel useful, even though I am not as productive as I used to be.* Or, *I still need to feel connected to my spouse even though now we are busier than ever.* Or, *I need to feel normal—to some extent—and that I am a part of life!* Or, *I need to make my needs a priority—perhaps for the first time in my life.*

# Engage in Acts of Selflessness

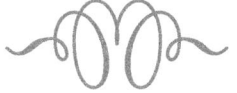

Selflessly helping another being is an act of powerful healing—especially when you are facing a cancer challenge and are preoccupied with worries surrounding your disease. In the space provided, explore ways you can engage with and provide help for those in need. For example, you could simply pray for others who are in need, drop off a family-sized meal to a struggling single parent, or volunteer your time to a worthy cause. Which opportunities to serve feel most comfortable and doable for you?

# Explore the Rewards of Serving Others

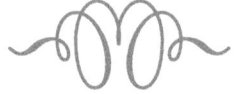

Don't be surprised if volunteering your time or going out of your way to help out someone else gives you a surprising burst of energy and joy. In the space provided, explore how being of service to others relates to shifting your vibrational frequency and impacts your immune system. Describe how you feel physically and emotionally both before and after engaging in a selfless act of kindness.

# You Really *Are* What You Eat!

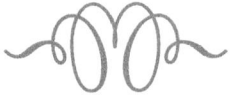

Viewing nutrition—the foods and beverages we consume—as *medicine* revolutionizes the way you think about your food and allows you to make powerful new choices that contribute to your overall wellness. *An Inside Job* addresses several dietary philosophies aimed at helping you understand how your food and drink choices may help you fight cancer. What changes do you see yourself making regarding adding and deleting foods from your diet? What feels doable for you? What changes in your shopping and lifestyle do you feel you can make? Write your reflections in the space below.

# Intentionally Nourishing Your Temple

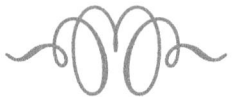

There are many aspects you can integrate into your life that will enable you to live joyfully. You can cultivate gratitude by focusing on your blessings, keeping a gratitude journal, or by affirming the gratitude you feel; you can treat your body with unconditional love by curtailing excessive stress, alcohol, and chemicals; you can enjoy a small indulgence like a bubble bath, a funny television show, a night in with a good book, or listen to music that makes you happy. When fighting cancer, it is important to purposefully care for your body and soul so your spirit is joyful and dwells in a state of higher vibrations. In the space provided, list the steps you will take to fill your life with ongoing joy and peace. Also, please note any stumbling blocks you anticipate and how you see yourself handling them!

# Your Thoughts Compose Your Reality

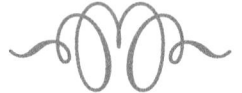

Consider the following thought: *Life is a journey, made of a fabric woven by your thoughts and feelings.* In the space provided, reflect on the value of focusing on thoughts and feelings that raise your vibrations—versus thoughts, focal points, and feelings that lower your vibrations. Here are some aspects that may raise your vibrations: your life passion, whatever brings you joy, positive affirmations, your favorite music, humor, inspirational stories, etc.

# Getting Fine Is Hard

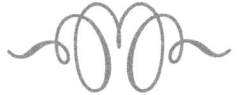

For many, a cancer diagnosis is an opportunity to unlock artistry that may have otherwise remained dormant. *An Inside Job* features two poems written by two-time cancer survivor Judy Lang: *Getting Fine Is Hard* and *One Year Later: A Cancer Survivor*. What messages do you take from Judy Lang's poems? What aspects of the poems move and touch you regarding your own cancer challenge?

# Be Selective in Choosing Your Medical Team and Protocol

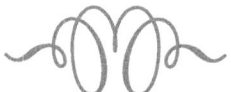

When facing cancer, it is important to choose healers who not only possess technical skill but intuition as well. You need to be able to trust and be comfortable with your healing team, as well as to feel respected by them. Finally, it is important to seek healers who are open to an integrative approach to your overall protocol. This enables you to approach healing on several levels: physical, emotional, mental, and spiritual—in such a way that you feel empowered, confident, and comfortable. Additionally, an integrative approach marries eastern and western techniques to expedite the healing of mind, body, and spirit. It revolves around your being in a better place energetically, to expedite the work of your immune system. Such an approach also addresses the need to make necessary lifestyle changes, including changes in nutrition, exercise, and your perspective about life as well as your illness. What guidelines would you recommend to a loved one (or for yourself) recently diagnosed with cancer? Does your current doctor meet these guidelines?

# Caring for the Whole Person

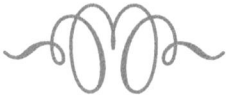

What does integrative medicine mean to you? What aspects of integrative medicine can you incorporate into your daily routine along your cancer journey? In addition to chemotherapy, radiation, and immunotherapy, many diagnosed with cancer are integrating other healing aspects into their treatment protocols. These include: yoga classes, tai chi, qigong, acupuncture sessions, energy medicine sessions, emotional code work (to release the vibrations of stored emotions), Reiki and Therapeutic Touch Sessions, and herbal supplementation. Additionally, consider enriching your treatment protocol by finding ways in which you can follow your passion and be of service to others. These activities are so powerful in enabling you to energetically shift to a higher vibration that they enormously bolster the immune system.

# Set the Stage for Healing with Your "Intention Statement"

After a cancer diagnosis, you will consider many options while deciding on your course of treatment. An important part of this process is to affirm a healing intention to guide you through the upcoming protocols. Before formulating your healing plan and beginning treatment, decide what your overarching intention will be. Write it in the space provided and refer to it throughout your treatment to invite in continued healing. For example, it helps to form your intention statement by seeing yourself experiencing the life you desire in the future, actually lived in the here and now. Say and intend the following: *I intend to live fully and joyfully (with my loved ones) both in the present and in the future. Well-being is my birthright. I intend to experience healing moment by moment, fully and joyfully. Healing is my birthright. I intend to be present for joy, love, and peace. I intend to receive all that I need to expedite my body's return to wholeness, balance, and harmony.*

_____

_____

_____

_____

# Intuition and Your Treatment Plan

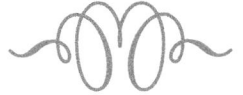

How might your intuition play a role in choosing your doctor, treatment, or routine? Do you tend to listen to your intuition? How can you tell when your intuition is speaking to you? Give examples recalling times you have and have not listened to your intuition—and the resulting consequences. Then, explore how you will continue using your intuition to make daily choices that support your healing.

# Finding Your Way with Integrative Healing

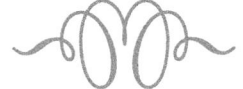

After reviewing the thoughts offered by the nine doctors in *An Inside Job*:

Comment on which of the doctors seemed to connect with you most deeply.

Ask yourself, *Which doctor most inspired and empowered me?*

Also, ask yourself, *What aspects of their recommendations and ways of thinking do I want to integrate into my own healing approach?*

Ask yourself, *What were the common themes in the doctors' thinking and philosophies regarding what is best for patients recently diagnosed with cancer?* Some examples might be: the value of an integrative approach, the significance of lifestyle, or the need to surrender fears and release negativity.

# Final Thoughts

My hope in writing *An Inside Job Companion: Making Healing Personal* is to enable you to recognize the beautiful, energetic being you are and discover that you have the inherent capacity to shift your own energetic vibrations to those that can help sustain a healthy immune system. This is the power with which you were born. Learning to harness your own energetic powers and gifts—including your breath, intuition, and imagination—enhances your sense of well-being, and helps create the balance, harmony, and peace you desire. This workbook is a space for you to explore and master the healing tools within, to develop perspectives that will allow you to experience greater joy and insight, and to nourish your soul and find spiritual healing.

Choosing the gift of love—unconditional love—for yourself and others is the key to all healing. This highest level of vibrations is adored by your body, composed of 60 trillion cells, and your immune system. So much of the journey is learning the art of loving yourself so deeply that you release and detach from whatever you have been vibrationally and energetically holding onto that your body knows is not good for you.

Bear in mind that healing occurs on many levels and in many ways. While no one can ever guarantee how and what type of healing will occur, know that *any* healing has everything to do with how you feel energetically. As you begin and end your day, I encourage you to affirm *I choose to be love, loving, and loved, and I am here for love and joy.* Also, choose to integrate the high vibrations of love, joy, and heartfelt appreciation and gratitude for your blessings into each and every moment of your life and relationships. Your mind, body, and spirit cherish these vibrations because they feel delicious and beautiful…and because they create peace, harmony, and balance for you. And this is what true healing is all about.

Blessings of peace and love, always.
—Susan

# About the Author

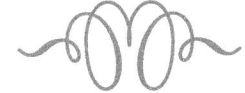

Susan Barbara Apollon is a Pennsylvania-licensed psychologist, as well as a cancer survivor and thriver. She has been in private practice since 1991 and specializes in grief, integrative oncology, and trauma. She is also an author, educator, and researcher of consciousness, mind, prayer, intuition, angels, energy, and healing.

Physicians refer their patients to Susan for assistance in healing their grief or meeting their cancer challenge. Susan's roots are in medicine. Her path and her approach, however, have enabled her to develop a unique perspective on healing—one that is based on an understanding that everything is energy and that energy is also medicine. With certification in Eden Energy Medicine and training in a number of energy modalities, as well as Energy Psychology, Susan shares with her patients her research findings concerning the primary factors that contribute to remission and healing. Her intention is to provide them with the wisdom and tools needed to achieve balance and wholeness, as well as to survive and thrive.

Susan has written a number of books. Her most recent title—which accompanies this workbook—is *An Inside Job: A Psychologist Shares Healing Wisdom for Your Cancer Journey*. Her other books include: *Touched by the Extraordinary (Book One); Touched by the Extraordinary, Book Two: Healing Stories of Love, Loss & Hope; Affirmations for Healing Mind, Body & Spirit*; and (coauthor) *Intuition Is Easy and Fun*. She is also the creator of several CDs, including: *Guided Meditation for Peace, Healing and Empowerment; Healing, Loving Imagery to Comfort and Soothe the Soul Challenged by Cancer; A Healing Meditation to Successfully Meet the Challenge of Cancer*; and *The Healing Power of Love*. Susan hopes this body of work will enable readers and listeners to appreciate the extraordinary spiritual implications of their journey with grief and/or cancer.

Susan loves sharing her passion for healing and the extraordinary (including miracles, the power of prayer, and angels). Her belief in the inherent healing wisdom and power within each of us, along with her unique blend of research and personal anecdotal material and stories, have helped many to shift and grow spiritually.

Her articles have appeared in national publications, including magazines, newspapers, and websites. Additionally, she has been a guest on numerous radio and television shows. She has conducted workshops, taught seminars, led healing retreats, and been asked to be a part of interfaith events.

Susan is honored to co-lead The GyniGirls, along with Dr. Amy Harvey. Being a part of this women's cancer support group nurtures her soul. Additionally, she enjoys speaking and sharing her research, as well as volunteering at a free monthly Energy Medicine Clinic.

Family, friends, and pets mean everything to Susan. When not engaged in research, writing, speaking, and her clinical work, she longs to be out in nature. What she loves most is being with her husband, to whom she has been married for 50 years, her children—especially her grandchildren—her cherished pets, and dear friends. She knows she is richly blessed.

# Book Susan Apollon to Speak to Your Organization or Group

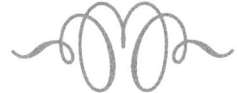

Susan Apollon speaks joyfully and passionately to hospital staffs and patients, medical students, college students, and other organizations and groups about everyone's ability to live full, satisfying lives, be happy, create their own miracles, and heal themselves. Often, she is honored to be asked to serve as a keynote speaker.

In addition, Susan conducts a rich variety of workshops and seminars that provide a blend of her contagious enthusiasm with her tried and true methods and interventions for energetic, physical, psychological and spiritual healing; empowerment; and creating a joyful and healthy life.

Susan is happy to speak and conduct interactive sessions on a variety of topics ranging from cancer, grief, integrative medicine, healing, love, near-death experiences, angels, prayers, and miracles. For a complete list of topics, please visit www.AnInsideJobForHealingCancer.com. Or call (215) 493-8434 for more information.